UNDERSTANDING, MANAGING, AND THRIVING WITH HYPOTHYROIDISM

Your Comprehensive Guide

Adams .U. Morris

TABLE OF CONTENTS

CHAPTER 1

Introduction To Hypothyroidism

Defining Hypothyroidism

Hypothyroidism is a medical condition that affects millions of people worldwide. To kickstart our journey into understanding this condition, let's begin with the basics. Hypothyroidism, often referred to as an underactive thyroid, occurs when the thyroid gland in your neck doesn't produce enough thyroid hormones to meet your body's needs. These hormones, called thyroxine (T4) and triiodothyronine (T3), play a crucial role in regulating your metabolism, energy production, and overall well-being.

The Prevalence of Hypothyroidism You might be surprised to learn just how common hypothyroidism is. It doesn't discriminate based on age, gender, or ethnicity. It can affect anyone, from children to the elderly. In fact, statistics show that hypothyroidism is more prevalent in women, especially as they get older. However, men and children are by no means immune.

The Thyroid's Role in the Body Now, let's delve into the thyroid gland itself. This butterfly-shaped gland, located at the base of your neck, may seem small, but it wields tremendous power. Its primary function is to produce and release thyroid hormones, which are essentially the body's internal regulators. Think of them as the conductors of a vast orchestra, directing every cell in your body to perform harmoniously. When the thyroid orchestra falls out of tune, as in hypothyroidism, it can have profound effects on your overall health.

Hypothyroidism's Impact on Health Hypothyroidism is like a disruptive player in this delicate orchestra. When there aren't enough thyroid hormones, your body's processes begin to slow down. This slowdown can manifest in a wide range of symptoms, affecting virtually every system in your body.

Imagine feeling fatigued all the time, despite getting enough sleep. Picture unexplained weight gain, even when you're watching your diet. Consider the emotional toll of feeling depressed, anxious, or irritable for no apparent reason.

These are just a few of the ways hypothyroidism can impact your life.

Physical symptoms can be equally challenging. You might notice your hair thinning, your skin becoming dry and pale, and your nails becoming brittle. Constipation, joint pain, and muscle weakness can become daily battles. Perhaps most distressing, your menstrual cycle may become irregular, or you might experience fertility issues.

Moreover, undiagnosed or untreated hypothyroidism can lead to serious complications over time. These can include heart problems, elevated cholesterol levels, and, in severe cases, a life-threatening condition called myxedema coma.

Given the far-reaching effects of hypothyroidism, early detection and management are crucial. Unfortunately, because its symptoms can mimic those of many other conditions, diagnosis can be challenging. That's why awareness and understanding are vital.

This chapter sets the stage for our exploration of hypothyroidism. We've defined the condition, looked at its prevalence, and delved into the thyroid gland's vital role in our bodies. We've also touched on the wide-ranging impact of hypothyroidism on health, emphasizing the importance of early recognition and treatment.

As we continue our journey through the remaining chapters, we'll dive deeper into the intricacies of hypothyroidism. We'll explore its causes, the diagnostic process, various treatment options, and the role of nutrition, lifestyle, and wellness in managing this condition. Finally, we'll conclude with a message of hope, encouraging individuals with hypothyroidism to take charge of their health and seek the support and resources they need to live well with this condition.

CHAPTER 2

Understanding the Thyroid Gland

In this chapter, we will delve deep into the thyroid gland itself, exploring its anatomy, function, and the vital hormones it produces. Understanding the intricacies of this tiny but powerful organ is essential for comprehending hypothyroidism and its impact on the body.

Anatomy of the Thyroid Gland

Picture a small, butterfly-shaped gland situated in the front of your neck, just below the Adam's apple. That's the thyroid gland. It may seem unassuming, but it plays a monumental role in your health.

The thyroid gland is comprised of two lobes, one on each side of your windpipe, joined by a narrow band of tissue called the isthmus. This arrangement is what gives it the butterfly-like appearance. The thyroid's location is crucial because it's nestled in a region rich with blood vessels, making it highly efficient at its job.

Function of the Thyroid Gland

The thyroid gland is essentially your body's metabolic regulator. It's responsible for producing thyroid hormones, primarily thyroxine (T4) and triiodothyronine (T3), which are released into your bloodstream. Think of these hormones as messengers that convey instructions to nearly every cell in your body.

Thyroid Hormones and Their Functions

Now, let's dive into what these thyroid hormones actually do:

1. **T4 (Thyroxine):** This hormone is like a precursor. It's produced in greater quantities by the thyroid gland and serves as a reservoir for T3. T4 gets converted into T3 as needed by your cells. T4's primary role is to provide a steady supply of T3 for your body to use when required.

2. **T3 (Triiodothyronine):** T3 is the active form of thyroid hormone. It's the one that directly influences

your body's metabolism. T3
stimulates the cells to
produce energy, regulate
body temperature, and
maintain heart rate. It plays
a key role in ensuring that
your body's metabolic
processes function
efficiently.

The Hypothalamus-Pituitary-Thyroid Axis

The regulation of thyroid
hormones is an intricate dance
involving the hypothalamus, the
pituitary gland, and the thyroid
gland. This axis is crucial for

maintaining hormonal balance in your body.

- **Hypothalamus:** This region in your brain acts as the control center. When it senses that thyroid hormone levels are low, it releases thyrotropin-releasing hormone (TRH).

- **Pituitary Gland:** Located at the base of your brain, the pituitary gland receives the message from the hypothalamus and responds by secreting thyroid-stimulating hormone (TSH).

- **Thyroid Gland:** Upon receiving the signal from the pituitary gland, the thyroid gland gets to work. It releases T4 and T3 in response to the elevated TSH levels.

This feedback loop ensures that your body maintains a stable level of thyroid hormones, allowing for optimal metabolic function.

Common Causes of Hypothyroidism

Now that we have a solid understanding of how the thyroid gland functions when everything is in balance, let's explore what can go wrong. There are several common causes of hypothyroidism:

1. **Autoimmune Thyroiditis (Hashimoto's Disease):** This is the most frequent cause of hypothyroidism in developed countries. It occurs when the body's immune system mistakenly attacks and damages the thyroid gland, reducing its ability to produce hormones.

2. **Thyroid Surgery or Radiation Therapy:** In some cases, surgical removal

of the thyroid gland or radiation treatment for conditions like thyroid cancer can result in hypothyroidism.

3. **Medications:** Certain medications, such as lithium and amiodarone, can interfere with thyroid hormone production.

4. **Iodine Deficiency:** While rare in regions with sufficient dietary iodine, a lack of this essential mineral can lead to hypothyroidism.

5. **Congenital Hypothyroidism:** Some individuals are born with an

underactive thyroid gland due to genetic factors or issues during fetal development.

6. **Pituitary or Hypothalamus Disorders:** Dysfunction in the pituitary gland or hypothalamus can disrupt the delicate balance of the hypothalamus-pituitary-thyroid axis, leading to hypothyroidism.

Understanding these causes will be crucial as we continue our exploration of hypothyroidism in the subsequent chapters. We'll delve into the signs and symptoms of this condition, how it's diagnosed, and the various treatment options available to help individuals with hypothyroidism regain control of their health and well-being.

CHAPTER 3

Signs and Symptoms

In this chapter, we will thoroughly explore the myriad signs and symptoms associated with hypothyroidism. Understanding these cues is essential for early detection and effective management of the condition.

Recognizing the Signs and Symptoms

Hypothyroidism is often called a "silent" condition because its symptoms can be subtle and easily mistaken for other health issues. However, over time, these symptoms can become more pronounced and have a profound impact on your overall well-being.

1. **Fatigue:** Overwhelming tiredness is one of the hallmark symptoms of hypothyroidism. You may find it increasingly difficult to summon the energy for even routine activities. This fatigue often persists, even after a full night's sleep.

2. **Weight Gain:** Unexplained weight gain is another common symptom. The

slowed metabolism associated with hypothyroidism can cause you to gain weight or make it difficult to lose weight, even when you're maintaining a healthy diet and exercise routine.

3. **Cold Intolerance:** Hypothyroidism can disrupt your body's temperature regulation, making you more sensitive to cold. You might feel cold all the time, even in warm environments.

4. **Dry Skin and Hair:** Your skin may become dry and flaky, and your hair can

become brittle and thin. Nails can also become weak and break easily.

5. **Depression and Mood Changes:** Changes in thyroid hormone levels can affect brain function and mood. Many individuals with hypothyroidism report feelings of depression, irritability, and anxiety.

6. **Memory and Concentration Issues:** Some people with hypothyroidism experience cognitive difficulties, such as forgetfulness and difficulty concentrating.

7. **Constipation:** Sluggish digestive processes are common in hypothyroidism, leading to chronic constipation.

8. **Menstrual Irregularities:** Women with hypothyroidism may experience irregular menstrual cycles, heavy periods, or even fertility issues.

9. **Muscle and Joint Pain:** Muscle weakness and joint pain can be bothersome symptoms. These issues can make everyday tasks more challenging.

10. **Hoarseness and Swelling in the Neck:** As the thyroid gland enlarges in some cases, it can cause visible swelling in the neck, known as a goiter. This may lead to hoarseness and difficulty swallowing.

11. **Elevated Cholesterol Levels:** Hypothyroidism can increase cholesterol levels, potentially contributing to heart disease if left untreated.

12. **Slowed Heart Rate:** Your heart rate might slow down, leading to bradycardia, a

condition where the heart beats too slowly.

Subclinical vs. Clinical Hypothyroidism

It's important to mention that there are different forms of hypothyroidism. The symptoms mentioned above primarily pertain to clinical hypothyroidism, where thyroid hormone levels are significantly low.

However, there's also a condition called subclinical hypothyroidism. In this milder form, the thyroid hormone levels are not as severely affected, and some individuals may experience very subtle or even no symptoms at all. Still, subclinical hypothyroidism should not be ignored, as it can progress to clinical hypothyroidism over time.

The Importance of Early Diagnosis

Given the diversity and subtlety of these symptoms, it's crucial to recognize the signs of hypothyroidism and seek medical attention if you suspect you may have this condition. Early diagnosis and treatment can significantly improve your quality of life and prevent potential complications.

Furthermore, because hypothyroidism shares symptoms with numerous other conditions, a comprehensive medical evaluation is necessary for accurate diagnosis. Doctors typically use blood tests to measure levels of thyroid hormones (TSH, T4, and T3) and antibodies associated with autoimmune thyroiditis (Hashimoto's disease) to confirm the diagnosis.

By understanding these signs and symptoms, you're better equipped to recognize when something might be amiss with your thyroid function. This awareness empowers you to seek the appropriate medical evaluation and take the necessary steps to manage hypothyroidism effectively.

As we continue through the subsequent chapters, we'll explore the diagnostic process in more detail, the various treatment options available, and the significance of lifestyle and dietary choices in managing this condition. Ultimately, the goal is to provide you with the knowledge and tools to reclaim your vitality and lead a fulfilling life despite hypothyroidism.

CHAPTER 4

Diagnosis and Testing

In this chapter, we'll delve into the diagnostic process for hypothyroidism, shedding light on the various tests and evaluations used by healthcare professionals to confirm this condition. Timely and accurate diagnosis is a crucial first step towards effective management.

The Diagnostic Process

Diagnosing hypothyroidism is a multi-step process that typically involves the following components:

1. **Medical History:** Your healthcare provider will begin by taking a thorough medical history. They will ask about your symptoms, family history of thyroid disorders, and any other relevant medical conditions or medications you're taking. This information helps in assessing your risk factors and guiding the diagnostic process.

2. **Physical Examination:** A physical examination is

often conducted, focusing on the neck area. The healthcare provider may palpate your thyroid gland for any enlargement (a goiter) or unusual nodules.

3. **Blood Tests:** Blood tests are the primary tools used to diagnose and monitor thyroid function. The key thyroid-related blood tests include:

    o **Thyroid-Stimulating Hormone (TSH):** This hormone, produced by the pituitary gland, stimulates the thyroid gland to produce T4 and T3. Elevated TSH levels can indicate an underactive thyroid (hypothyroidism).

- **Free Thyroxine (Free T4):** This test measures the level of unbound (free) T4 in your bloodstream. Low levels can indicate hypothyroidism.
- **Total Triiodothyronine (Total T3):** Though less commonly used than TSH and Free T4,

Total T3 measures the total amount of T3 in your blood. It can be helpful in some cases of thyroid disease diagnosis.

- **Thyroid Peroxidase Antibodies (TPOAb) and Thyroglobulin Antibodies (TgAb):** Elevated levels of these antibodies in your blood can indicate an autoimmune thyroid disorder, such as Hashimoto's disease.

4. **Imaging:** In some cases, imaging tests like thyroid ultrasound or a thyroid scan may be performed to assess the size and structure of the thyroid gland. These tests can help identify goiters or nodules.

5. **Fine-Needle Aspiration (FNA) Biopsy:** If nodules are found in the thyroid gland, an FNA biopsy may be recommended to determine whether they are cancerous or benign.

6. **Additional Tests:** Depending on your individual case and

symptoms, your healthcare provider may order additional tests to evaluate the impact of hypothyroidism on other aspects of your health. These can include lipid profiles to assess cholesterol levels, cardiac evaluations, and bone density tests, among others.

Interpreting Thyroid Function Test Results

Interpreting the results of thyroid function tests is a nuanced process. It's important to understand that reference ranges can vary between laboratories, so your healthcare provider will consider the specific reference ranges provided by the lab that conducted your tests.

- **TSH Levels:** Elevated TSH levels (above the reference range) are a primary indicator of hypothyroidism. Higher TSH indicates that the pituitary gland is working harder to stimulate the thyroid to produce more thyroid hormones because the body's levels are too low.
- **Free T4 Levels:** Low levels of Free T4, along with

elevated TSH, support the diagnosis of hypothyroidism. T4 is typically lower in hypothyroid patients because the thyroid gland is not producing enough of it.

Subclinical Hypothyroidism

In some cases, individuals may have mildly elevated TSH levels with normal Free T4 levels. This condition is known as subclinical hypothyroidism. It's essential to monitor individuals with subclinical hypothyroidism because it can progress to clinical hypothyroidism over time.

Understanding Autoimmune Thyroid Disorders

If your blood tests reveal elevated levels of thyroid antibodies, such as TPOAb and TgAb, this suggests an autoimmune thyroid disorder. The most common of these is Hashimoto's disease, which often leads to hypothyroidism.

The Role of Comprehensive Evaluation

Diagnosing hypothyroidism requires a comprehensive evaluation, considering not only thyroid function tests but also the patient's symptoms, medical history, and physical examination findings. Sometimes, symptoms and laboratory results may not align perfectly, making clinical judgment a crucial aspect of the diagnosis.

Special Considerations for Pregnancy

It's worth noting that pregnancy can complicate the interpretation of thyroid function tests. Thyroid hormones are essential for fetal development, and pregnancy can alter thyroid hormone levels. Pregnant individuals with hypothyroidism require special attention and management to ensure the health of both the mother and the baby.

In conclusion, the diagnostic process for hypothyroidism involves a combination of medical history, physical examination, blood tests, imaging, and, in some cases, biopsies. Interpreting the results of these tests requires expertise, as reference ranges can vary. Early and accurate diagnosis is vital because it paves the way for effective treatment and management.

In the subsequent chapters, we'll explore various treatment options for hypothyroidism, including conventional medications and alternative approaches. We'll also delve into the crucial role of nutrition, lifestyle modifications, and stress management in managing this condition effectively. Ultimately, our goal is to provide you with a comprehensive understanding of hypothyroidism and the tools to lead a fulfilling and healthy life despite its challenges.

CHAPTER 5

Treatment Options

In this chapter, we will explore the various treatment options available for managing hypothyroidism. Effective treatment can significantly improve the quality of life for individuals with this condition, and understanding the available approaches is essential.

Conventional Treatment with Synthetic Thyroid Hormones

The most common and widely accepted treatment for hypothyroidism is the use of synthetic thyroid hormones. The primary medication prescribed for this purpose is levothyroxine (often sold under brand names such as Synthroid or Levoxyl). Levothyroxine is a synthetic form of the thyroid hormone thyroxine (T4).

Here's how conventional treatment with levothyroxine works:

- **Supplementing Thyroid Hormones:** Since hypothyroidism is characterized by low thyroid hormone levels, levothyroxine is taken orally to provide the body with the hormone it needs.

- **Normalization of TSH Levels:** The goal of treatment is to bring the levels of thyroid-stimulating hormone (TSH) within the normal range. Elevated TSH levels indicate that the body is trying to stimulate the thyroid gland to produce more hormones. By restoring T4 levels with levothyroxine, TSH levels are usually brought back into the normal range.

- **Individualized Dosing:** The dosage of levothyroxine is individualized based on factors like age, weight, and the severity of hypothyroidism. It's crucial to follow your healthcare provider's recommended dosage and have regular follow-up appointments to fine-tune the treatment.

Effectiveness and Monitoring

Levothyroxine is highly effective in treating hypothyroidism when prescribed correctly. It generally produces noticeable improvements in symptoms such as fatigue, cold intolerance, and weight gain within a few weeks to a few months of starting treatment.

However, it's essential to monitor thyroid function regularly after starting treatment. This is done through blood tests to check TSH levels. The goal is to keep TSH levels within the normal range to maintain optimal thyroid function and symptom relief.

Alternative Thyroid Hormone Medications

While levothyroxine is the most commonly prescribed medication for hypothyroidism, there are alternative thyroid hormone medications available. Some individuals may not respond well to levothyroxine or may have specific preferences for other formulations. These alternative medications include:

1. **Liothyronine (T3):** This medication contains triiodothyronine (T3), the active form of thyroid hormone. It can be used alone or in combination with levothyroxine.

2. **Natural Desiccated Thyroid (NDT):** NDT is derived from the thyroid glands of animals (usually pigs) and contains both T3 and T4. It's often chosen by individuals who prefer a more natural approach.

3. **Combination T4/T3 Therapy:** Some patients may benefit from a combination of levothyroxine (T4) and liothyronine (T3) to achieve better symptom control.

Lifestyle Modifications and Hypothyroidism

While medication is the cornerstone of hypothyroidism treatment, lifestyle modifications can complement medical therapy and improve overall well-being. Here are some key lifestyle considerations:

1. **Diet:** A balanced diet with sufficient nutrients, particularly iodine and selenium, can support thyroid health. However, dietary changes should be made in consultation with a healthcare provider, as some foods can interfere with

thyroid medication absorption.

2. **Stress Management:** Chronic stress can impact thyroid function. Practices like meditation, yoga, and mindfulness can help reduce stress levels.

3. **Exercise:** Regular physical activity can boost metabolism and alleviate some hypothyroidism symptoms like fatigue and weight gain. Consult your healthcare provider before starting any new exercise regimen.

4. **Sleep:** Prioritize good sleep hygiene to ensure restful sleep, which is crucial for overall health, including thyroid function.

5. **Medication Timing:** Take thyroid medication as prescribed, and avoid taking it with foods or supplements that may interfere with its absorption, such as calcium or iron supplements.

6. **Avoiding Goitrogens:** Some foods, known as goitrogens, can interfere with thyroid function. These include cruciferous vegetables like broccoli and

cabbage. While it's generally not necessary to avoid these foods entirely, cooking or steaming them can reduce their goitrogenic effects.

Patient-Doctor Collaboration

Effective management of hypothyroidism requires ongoing collaboration between you and your healthcare provider. Regular follow-up appointments are essential to monitor your progress, adjust medication dosages as needed, and address any concerns or changes in symptoms.

It's crucial to communicate openly with your healthcare provider about your symptoms, lifestyle changes, and any side effects or concerns related to your medication. This collaborative approach ensures that your treatment plan remains tailored to your specific needs.

Conclusion

In this chapter, we've explored the primary treatment options for hypothyroidism, with a focus on conventional medication using synthetic thyroid hormones like levothyroxine. These medications are highly effective when prescribed and monitored correctly, allowing individuals with hypothyroidism to regain normal thyroid function and improve their quality of life.

We've also touched on alternative thyroid hormone medications, lifestyle modifications, and the importance of patient-doctor collaboration in achieving optimal outcomes. With the right treatment plan and ongoing support, individuals with hypothyroidism can lead healthy and fulfilling lives, managing their condition effectively.

CHAPTER 6

Managing Hypothyroidism Through Nutrition

In this chapter, we'll delve into the crucial role of nutrition in managing hypothyroidism. The food you eat can have a significant impact on your thyroid health and overall well-being, and understanding the relationship between nutrition and hypothyroidism is vital for effective management.

The Role of Diet in Thyroid Health

The thyroid gland relies on specific nutrients to produce thyroid hormones effectively. Therefore, maintaining a balanced diet is essential for supporting thyroid function. Here are some key considerations:

1. **Iodine:** Iodine is a critical component of thyroid hormones. The thyroid gland combines iodine with tyrosine (an amino acid) to create thyroid hormones. Insufficient iodine intake can lead to thyroid

dysfunction. However, iodine deficiency is relatively rare in regions with access to iodized salt and a varied diet.

- o *Dietary Sources:* Iodine-rich foods include seafood (e.g., fish and seaweed), dairy products, and iodized salt.

2. **Selenium:** Selenium is another essential mineral for thyroid health. It is a component of enzymes that help convert T4 (inactive thyroid hormone) into T3 (active thyroid hormone).

- *Dietary Sources:* Selenium-rich foods include Brazil nuts, sunflower seeds, fish, and lean meats.

3. **Zinc:** Zinc plays a role in thyroid hormone production and the conversion of T4 to T3.

   - *Dietary Sources:* Zinc can be found in foods like oysters, beef, poultry, and whole grains.

4. **Iron:** Iron is needed for proper thyroid function and is essential for the enzymes that convert T4 to T3.

o   *Dietary Sources:* Good sources of iron include lean meats, poultry, fish, beans, and fortified cereals.

5. **Vitamins:** Certain vitamins, particularly vitamins A, D, and B12, are important for thyroid health and overall metabolism.

o   *Dietary Sources:* Foods rich in these vitamins include liver, fatty fish, eggs, dairy products, and fortified cereals.

Hypothyroidism and Diet

While a balanced diet that provides essential nutrients is generally beneficial for thyroid health, some dietary considerations specifically apply to individuals with hypothyroidism:

1. **Soy and Cruciferous Vegetables:** Soy and cruciferous vegetables like broccoli, cauliflower, cabbage, and kale contain compounds known as goitrogens. In large amounts, goitrogens can interfere with thyroid hormone production. However, cooking these

foods can help neutralize their goitrogenic effects, making them safe to consume in moderation.

2. **Fiber:** Hypothyroidism can sometimes lead to constipation, and increasing fiber intake can be beneficial. However, some sources of dietary fiber, like bran, may interfere with the absorption of thyroid medication if consumed too close to taking the medication. It's advisable to separate medication and high-fiber meals by a few hours.

3. **Calcium and Iron Supplements:** If you take calcium or iron supplements, be cautious about taking them at the same time as your thyroid medication. These minerals can interfere with the absorption of thyroid hormones, so it's best to take them at separate times of the day.

Nutritional Deficiencies Common in Hypothyroidism

Hypothyroidism can lead to specific nutritional deficiencies, partly due to the condition's effects on digestion and metabolism. These deficiencies may exacerbate hypothyroidism symptoms and should be addressed:

1. **Vitamin D:** Hypothyroidism has been associated with lower levels of vitamin D. Adequate vitamin D is important for overall health and may play a role in thyroid function.

2. **B Vitamins:** Deficiencies in B vitamins, particularly B12 and folate, can occur in individuals with hypothyroidism. These

vitamins are important for energy metabolism and overall well-being.

3. **Iron:** Chronic inflammation often seen in hypothyroidism can lead to anemia, which is characterized by low iron levels. Iron is crucial for carrying oxygen in the blood and supporting overall energy levels.

4. **Selenium:** Some individuals with hypothyroidism may have low selenium levels, which can impair thyroid function.

Addressing these deficiencies through dietary changes or supplementation, under the guidance of a healthcare provider, can improve thyroid function and overall health.

Meal Planning and Dietary Strategies for Hypothyroidism

If you have hypothyroidism, it's essential to maintain a balanced and nutritious diet that supports thyroid health. Here are some meal planning and dietary strategies to consider:

1. **Balanced Macronutrients:** Ensure your diet includes a balance of carbohydrates, proteins, and healthy fats. This can help stabilize blood sugar levels and maintain energy levels throughout the day.

2. **Regular Meals:** Aim to eat regular meals and snacks to avoid spikes and crashes in blood sugar levels, which can affect energy and mood.

3. **Hydration:** Drink plenty of water to stay well-hydrated. Dehydration can exacerbate some hypothyroidism symptoms.

4. **Limit Processed Foods:** Minimize the consumption of highly processed and sugary foods, which can lead to inflammation and energy fluctuations.

5. **Moderate Alcohol and Caffeine:** Excessive alcohol and caffeine consumption can disrupt sleep and affect energy levels. Limiting these substances may help manage symptoms.

6. **Monitor Iodine Intake:** In regions with sufficient dietary iodine, it's generally not necessary to increase iodine intake. Excessive

iodine can actually worsen thyroid function in some cases.

7. **Consult a Dietitian:** Consider consulting a registered dietitian or nutritionist with expertise in thyroid health. They can help you create a personalized meal plan that meets your nutritional needs while managing hypothyroidism.

Conclusion

Nutrition plays a pivotal role in managing hypothyroidism. A well-balanced diet that provides essential nutrients like iodine, selenium, and vitamins is crucial for supporting thyroid function and overall health. Understanding the specific dietary considerations for hypothyroidism, such as managing goitrogenic foods and separating medication from certain nutrients, is essential for effective management.

Additionally, addressing nutritional deficiencies that often accompany hypothyroidism can alleviate symptoms and improve overall well-being. Meal planning and dietary strategies can help individuals with hypothyroidism maintain stable energy levels, manage weight, and optimize thyroid function.

In the subsequent chapters, we will continue our exploration of hypothyroidism by delving into lifestyle modifications, exercise, and stress management, all of which are essential components of a holistic approach to managing this condition effectively.

CHAPTER 7

Lifestyle Modifications for Hypothyroidism Management

In this chapter, we'll explore the significant role that lifestyle modifications play in effectively managing hypothyroidism. While medication is a cornerstone of treatment, making specific lifestyle changes can significantly improve your overall well-being and thyroid function.

The Impact of Lifestyle on Hypothyroidism

Hypothyroidism affects various aspects of your life, from energy levels to metabolism and mood. Incorporating positive lifestyle changes can help mitigate the impact of this condition, reduce symptoms, and enhance your overall quality of life. Here are some key lifestyle modifications to consider:

1. Stress Management:

Stress can have a profound impact on thyroid health. Chronic stress triggers the release of cortisol, a hormone that can interfere with thyroid function. Stress can also exacerbate symptoms like fatigue and mood swings. Therefore, managing stress is a crucial aspect of hypothyroidism management.

Stress Reduction Techniques:

- **Meditation and Mindfulness:** These practices can help you stay present, reduce anxiety, and manage stress more effectively.
- **Yoga:** Yoga combines physical postures, breathing exercises, and meditation to promote relaxation and reduce stress.
- **Deep Breathing Exercises:** Simple deep-

breathing exercises can calm your nervous system and reduce stress levels.

- **Adequate Sleep:** Prioritize sleep hygiene to ensure restful sleep, which can improve your ability to handle stress.

2. Regular Exercise:

Exercise can boost metabolism, improve mood, and increase energy levels—all of which can be especially beneficial for individuals with hypothyroidism. However, it's essential to choose an exercise routine that aligns with your fitness level and takes into account your individual health considerations.

Exercise Options:

- **Aerobic Exercise:** Activities like walking, jogging, swimming, or cycling can help increase cardiovascular fitness and boost energy levels.

- **Strength Training:** Resistance exercises with weights or resistance bands can help build muscle mass and support metabolic function.

- **Yoga and Tai Chi:** These practices combine physical

activity with relaxation techniques, making them suitable options for stress reduction.

It's crucial to consult your healthcare provider before starting a new exercise program, especially if you have other health conditions or concerns.

3. Diet and Nutrition:

As discussed in the previous chapter, diet plays a vital role in thyroid health. Maintaining a balanced diet that provides essential nutrients can support thyroid function and overall well-being.

Nutrition Considerations:

- **Balanced Macronutrients:** Ensure your diet includes a balance of carbohydrates, proteins, and healthy fats to stabilize blood sugar levels and maintain energy throughout the day.

- **Hydration:** Drink plenty of water to stay well-hydrated. Dehydration can exacerbate some hypothyroidism symptoms.

- **Limit Processed Foods:** Minimize highly processed and sugary foods, which can lead to inflammation and energy fluctuations.

- **Iodine Awareness:** In regions with sufficient dietary iodine, it's generally not necessary to increase iodine intake. Excessive iodine can worsen thyroid function in some cases.

- **Consult a Dietitian:** Consider working with a registered dietitian or nutritionist with expertise in thyroid health to create a personalized meal plan.

4. Sleep Hygiene:

Sleep is essential for overall health, and individuals with hypothyroidism may be more prone to sleep disturbances. Poor sleep can exacerbate fatigue and other symptoms.

Sleep Hygiene Tips:

- **Maintain a Consistent Sleep Schedule:** Go to bed and wake up at the same times each day, even on weekends.
- **Create a Relaxing Bedtime Routine:** Engage in calming activities before

bedtime, such as reading or taking a warm bath.

- **Create a Comfortable Sleep Environment:** Ensure your bedroom is conducive to sleep by keeping it dark, quiet, and at a comfortable temperature.

- **Limit Screen Time:** Reduce exposure to screens (phones, computers, TVs) before bedtime, as the blue light emitted can interfere with sleep.

- **Limit Stimulants:** Avoid caffeine and nicotine close to bedtime, as they can disrupt sleep.

5. Mind-Body Practices:

Mind-body practices encompass a range of techniques that promote relaxation and improve mental well-being. These practices can be particularly helpful for managing stress and improving overall quality of life with hypothyroidism.

Mind-Body Techniques:

- **Meditation:** Meditation involves focusing the mind on a particular object, thought, or activity to train attention and awareness. It can help reduce stress and improve emotional well-being.

- **Biofeedback:** Biofeedback is a therapeutic technique that helps individuals gain control over physiological functions such as heart rate and muscle tension. It can be useful for managing stress and anxiety.

- **Acupuncture:** Acupuncture involves the insertion of thin needles into specific points on the body. Some individuals with hypothyroidism have found acupuncture to be helpful in managing symptoms.

- **Relaxation Exercises:** Simple relaxation exercises, such as progressive muscle relaxation or guided imagery, can help reduce stress and improve sleep.

6. Supportive Therapies:

In addition to lifestyle modifications, some individuals with hypothyroidism find complementary and alternative therapies beneficial in managing their condition. These therapies should be used in conjunction with, not as a replacement for, conventional medical treatment. Some of these therapies include:

- **Chiropractic Care:** Chiropractic adjustments can help manage musculoskeletal symptoms often associated with hypothyroidism, such as joint and muscle pain.

- **Massage Therapy:** Massage can relieve muscle tension, reduce stress, and improve circulation.

- **Herbal Supplements:** Some herbal supplements, such as ashwagandha and guggul, are believed to support thyroid function. However, it's essential to consult with a healthcare provider before using any supplements, as they can interact with medications.

Conclusion

Lifestyle modifications are a crucial component of managing hypothyroidism effectively. By incorporating stress management techniques, regular exercise, a balanced diet, proper sleep hygiene, and mind-body practices, you can alleviate symptoms, improve energy levels, and enhance your overall well-being.

It's important to approach lifestyle modifications in consultation with your healthcare provider, especially if you have other health conditions or specific concerns related to hypothyroidism. A collaborative approach that combines lifestyle changes with appropriate medical treatment offers the best chance for individuals with hypothyroidism to lead healthy and fulfilling lives.

CHAPTER 8

Thriving with Hypothyroidism - Long-Term Strategies for Well-Being

In this final chapter, we will explore long-term strategies for thriving with hypothyroidism. Managing this condition isn't just about symptom relief; it's about achieving a fulfilling and healthy life. We'll discuss maintaining consistency in your treatment, setting realistic goals, finding support, and maintaining a positive outlook on your journey with hypothyroidism.

1. Consistency in Treatment:

Consistency in your treatment plan is essential for effectively managing hypothyroidism over the long term. Here are some key aspects to consider:

- **Medication Adherence:** Continue taking your prescribed thyroid medication as directed by your healthcare provider. Skipping doses or discontinuing medication can lead to symptom recurrence.

- **Regular Monitoring:** Schedule regular follow-up appointments to monitor your thyroid function. Your healthcare provider will adjust your medication dosage as needed to keep your thyroid hormone levels within the optimal range.

- **Lifestyle Modifications:** Maintain the lifestyle changes you've incorporated, such as stress management techniques, exercise routines, and dietary choices. Consistency in these areas can help prevent symptom flare-ups.

2. Setting Realistic Goals:

Living with hypothyroidism means managing a chronic condition. It's essential to set realistic goals and expectations for yourself. Here are some considerations:

- **Energy Levels:** Understand that you may have days when fatigue is more pronounced. Plan your activities accordingly and prioritize rest when needed.
- **Weight Management:** Achieving and maintaining a

healthy weight is possible with hypothyroidism, but it may require patience and adjustments to your diet and exercise routine. Avoid extreme diets or exercise regimens and focus on sustainable changes.

- **Symptom Control:** While thyroid medication can alleviate many symptoms, some may persist or fluctuate. Be patient with yourself and work closely with your healthcare provider to address ongoing symptoms.

- **Emotional Well-Being:** Managing stress and mood is an ongoing process. Set small, achievable goals for maintaining emotional well-being, such as practicing relaxation techniques and seeking support when needed.

3. Finding Support:

Living with hypothyroidism can be challenging at times, and having a support system can make a significant difference. Here are ways to find support:

- **Healthcare Provider:** Maintain open communication with your healthcare provider. Share your concerns, questions, and any changes in your symptoms. They can provide guidance and adjustments to your treatment plan.

- **Support Groups:** Joining a support group for individuals with thyroid conditions can be highly beneficial. These groups provide a platform to connect with others who understand what you're going through and can offer practical advice and emotional support.

- **Friends and Family:** Educate your close friends and family members about hypothyroidism so they can better understand your needs and offer support when necessary.

- **Mental Health Professionals:** If you experience persistent mood changes or emotional challenges, consider consulting a mental health professional. Therapy or counseling can be highly effective in managing emotional aspects of hypothyroidism.

4. Maintaining a Positive Outlook:

A positive outlook can significantly impact your experience with hypothyroidism. Here are ways to foster a positive mindset:

- **Education:** Continue learning about hypothyroidism and its management. Understanding your condition empowers you to take an active role in your health.

- **Gratitude:** Focus on the aspects of your life that bring you joy and gratitude. Practicing gratitude can help shift your perspective and improve your overall well-being.

- **Self-Compassion:** Be kind and patient with yourself. Managing a chronic condition is a journey with ups and downs, and it's okay to acknowledge your limitations and seek support when needed.

- **Holistic Approach:** Consider a holistic approach to your well-being, addressing physical, emotional, and spiritual aspects of your life. Engage in activities that bring you joy and fulfillment.

- **Life Balance:** Strive for balance in your life. Prioritize self-care and ensure you have time for relaxation, hobbies, and spending time with loved ones.

5. Staying Informed:

Stay informed about advances in thyroid health research and treatment options. Medical knowledge and technology are continually evolving, and new approaches to managing hypothyroidism may emerge. Discuss any new treatment options or research findings with your healthcare provider to determine if they are relevant to your care.

6. **Advocating for Yourself:

Become an advocate for your own health. If you ever feel that your symptoms are not adequately managed or that your treatment plan needs adjustment, communicate your concerns to your healthcare provider. Your

active involvement in your care
can lead to better outcomes.

CONCLUSION

Hypothyroidism is a chronic condition that requires long-term management, but it should not prevent you from leading a fulfilling and healthy life. By maintaining consistency in your treatment, setting realistic goals, finding support, and maintaining a positive outlook, you can thrive with hypothyroidism.

Remember that you are not alone in this journey. Support is available from healthcare professionals, support groups, friends, and family. Continue to educate yourself about hypothyroidism and its management, stay informed about new developments, and advocate for your health when necessary.

With the right treatment, lifestyle modifications, and support, individuals with hypothyroidism can lead vibrant and fulfilling lives. This final chapter marks the beginning of your journey to thriving with hypothyroidism, armed with knowledge and strategies to live your best life despite the challenges posed by this condition.

In conclusion, the journey through the eight chapters of this book has been a comprehensive exploration of hypothyroidism, a condition that affects millions of lives worldwide. From understanding the basics of thyroid function to learning about diagnosis, treatment options, and lifestyle management, we've covered the essential aspects of living with and managing hypothyroidism.

Hypothyroidism is a condition that requires ongoing attention and care. It can bring its challenges, including fatigue, weight fluctuations, mood changes, and more. However, armed with knowledge and a proactive approach, individuals can navigate these challenges and thrive.

The key takeaways from this book can be summarized as follows:

1. **Understanding Your Thyroid:** The thyroid is a small but powerful gland that plays a vital role in regulating your body's metabolism and overall health. Hypothyroidism occurs when this gland doesn't produce enough

thyroid hormones, leading to a range of symptoms.

2. **Recognizing Symptoms:** Hypothyroidism can manifest in various ways, from fatigue and weight gain to depression and cold intolerance. Being aware of these symptoms is crucial for early diagnosis.

3. **Diagnosis and Testing:** Proper diagnosis involves a combination of medical history, physical examination, and thyroid function tests. These tests, including TSH, Free T4, and antibodies, help healthcare

providers confirm and manage hypothyroidism.

4. **Treatment Options:** Conventional treatment for hypothyroidism often involves synthetic thyroid hormone replacement, such as levothyroxine. Alternative treatments and lifestyle modifications can also play a role in managing the condition effectively.

5. **Nutrition Matters:** A balanced diet rich in essential nutrients, such as iodine, selenium, and vitamins, is essential for supporting thyroid health.

Understanding the impact of certain foods and nutrients on thyroid function can help individuals make informed dietary choices.

6. **Lifestyle Modifications:** Stress management, regular exercise, quality sleep, and mind-body practices are powerful tools for managing hypothyroidism. Incorporating these strategies into your daily life can lead to better symptom control and overall well-being.

7. **Long-Term Thriving:** Consistency in treatment,

setting realistic goals, finding support, maintaining a positive outlook, staying informed, and advocating for your health are essential for thriving with hypothyroidism over the long term.

This book has aimed to provide not only knowledge but also empowerment. You now have the tools to understand your condition, collaborate effectively with healthcare providers, and make informed decisions about your health.

While living with hypothyroidism can present challenges, it's important to remember that you are not defined by your condition. With proper management, support, and a positive mindset, you can lead a fulfilling life, pursuing your goals and dreams.

Hypothyroidism is just one aspect of your life; it doesn't define who you are. Use the information in this book as a guide on your journey to better health and well-being. Whether you are recently diagnosed or have been living with hypothyroidism for some time, know that you have the resilience and strength to thrive.

As you move forward, continue to seek knowledge, explore treatment options, embrace a healthy lifestyle, and surround yourself with a supportive network of friends, family, and healthcare professionals. Remember, you are not alone on this journey, and there is a world of possibilities waiting for you beyond your diagnosis.

With determination, self-compassion, and the strategies outlined in this book, you can face the challenges of hypothyroidism with confidence and lead a vibrant, fulfilling life. Your journey to thriving starts now.